Diabetes
Sustenance

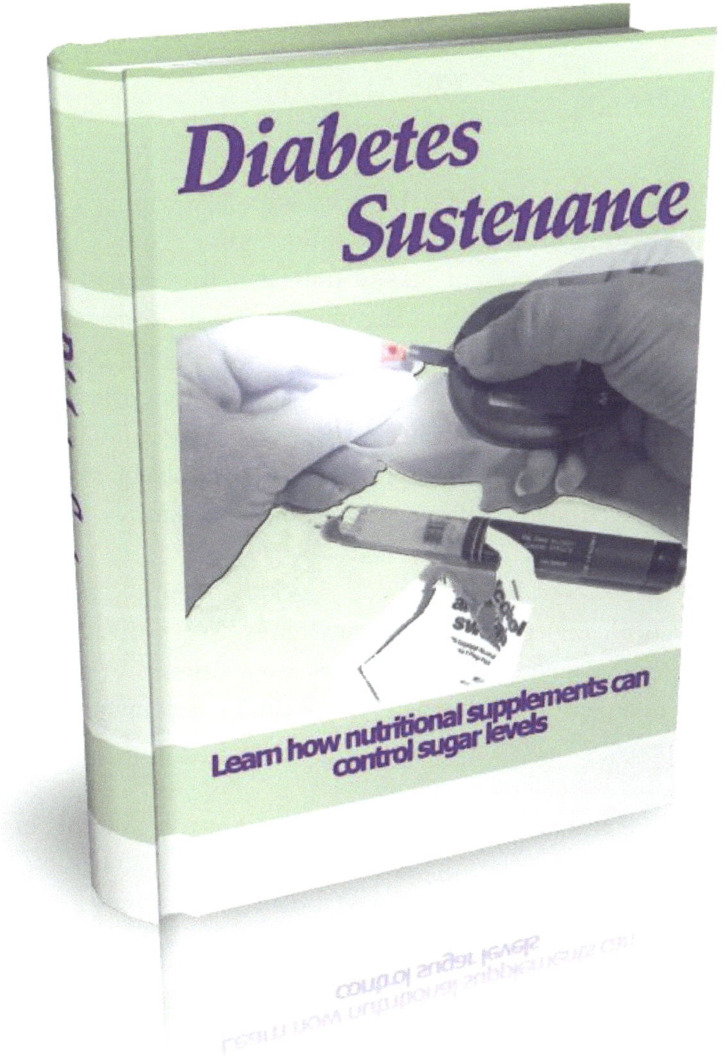

Learn how nutritional supplements can control sugar levels

Terms and Conditions

LEGAL NOTICE

The Publisher has strived to be as accurate and complete as possible in the creation of this report, notwithstanding the fact that he does not warrant or represent at any time that the contents within are accurate due to the rapidly changing nature of the Internet.

While all attempts have been made to verify information provided in this publication, the Publisher assumes no responsibility for errors, omissions, or contrary interpretation of the subject matter herein. Any perceived slights of specific persons, peoples, or organizations are unintentional.

In practical advice books, like anything else in life, there are no guarantees of income made. Readers are cautioned to reply on their own judgment about their individual circumstances to act accordingly.

This book is not intended for use as a source of legal, business, accounting or financial advice. All readers are advised to seek services of competent professionals in legal, business, accounting and finance fields.

You are encouraged to print this book for easy reading.

Table Of Contents

Foreword

Diabetes is already a fairly complicated medical condition and to further confuses the patient with a variety of nutritional information that might not even help and would have rather disastrous results. Get all the info you need here.

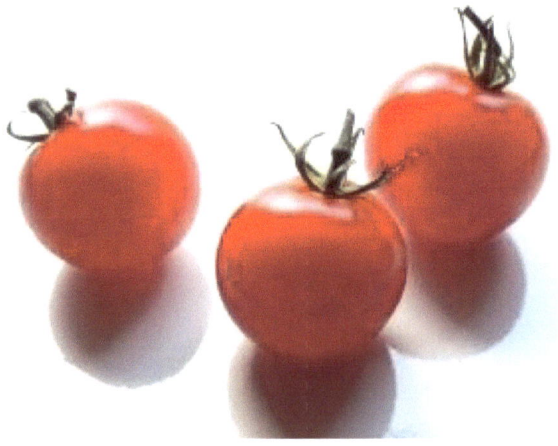

Diabetes Sustenance

Learn how nutritional supplements can control sugar levels

Chapter 1:

Principles of Diabetes Nutrition

Synopsis

Most diabetic patients are unaware of the extent the nutrition taken benefits or creates side effect for them. Therefore there is a need to ensure all nutritional supplements are taken with the approval of the consulting physician.

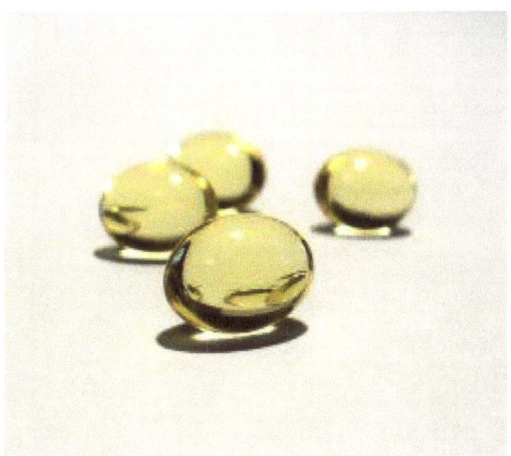

Nutrition

It is hoped that with the correct nutritional recommendation the patient will be able to attain and maintain optimal metabolic rates thus regulating the blood glucose levels to a normal range or at least to a more acceptable level.

These will the help to prevent or possibly reduce the risk of other related complication that diabetes bring on. Proper nutrition regiments for diabetes is also intended to ensure a lipid and lipoprotein profile is maintained to reduce the risk of macro vascular disease.

The nutrition choice is also designed to help create optimum blood pressure levels that will in turn help to reduce the risks of vascular diseases.

Nutrition regiments are also expected to help prevent and treat the chronic complications of the diabetic patient. The nutritional recommendations are modified to ensure a better lifestyle so that the diabetic patient can avoid possible obesity, dyslipidemia, cardiovascular diseases, hypertension and nephropathy. The nutritional intake would also require the patient to have an adequate amount of physical activity incorporated in to the lifestyle to ensure there is no possibility of the nutrient being retained in the system and build up to cause more problems.

It should be noted that there are several different categories and levels of diabetic problems, and as such each case may differ from the next. This would mean any nutrition diet plan prescribed has to be custom fitted to the individual patient's needs.

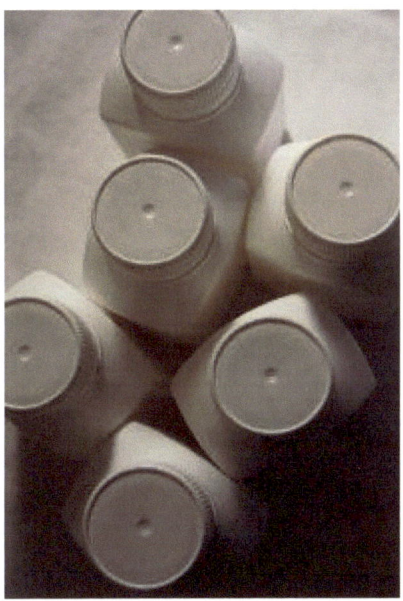

Chapter 2:

Your Diabetes Nutrition & Meal Plan

Synopsis

Although a diabetes food plan can be quite challenging to plan it does not have to be boring or tasteless, with at little guidance a diet plan that is both appetizing and nutritional can be drawn up.

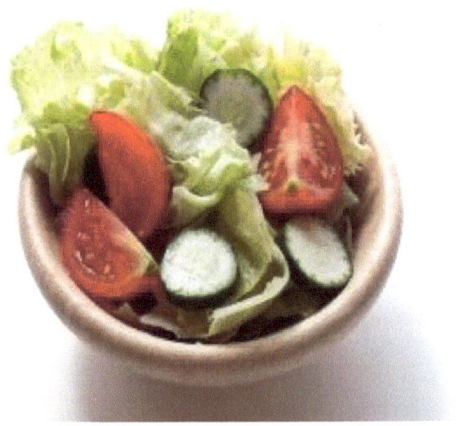

Diet Planning

A dietetic diet plan should ensure all the carbohydrates eaten during a daily diet is well spread out so as not to overwhelm the body's system. This is important as it helps to ensure the blood sugar levels are kept in control, therefore the need to keep track of what is being consumed.

The amount of carbs taken can also be regulated with the use of insulin and through exercise. Most diabetes also have to be concerned about the sodium content of the foods they consume as it can be have negative effects on the high blood pressure already present in most diabetic patients.

Therefore those with the added medical condition of hypertension would be weary of the sodium intake. For the diabetic with high levels of lipids the consumption of saturated fats, cholesterol and trans fats would be kept monitored.

When attempting to design a meal plan for a diabetic some points should be taken into consideration. These may include ensuring the calories intake is kept to about 10% to 20% from a protein source.

Meats such as chicken and beef should be considered over other choices. About 25% to 30% of the calories should come from fats however foods with saturated and trans fats should either be avoided or eaten in moderation. 50% to 60% of calories should come from carbohydrates. Eating lots of green and orange vegetables will help to keep the balance, and these would include carrots and broccoli. Eating brown rice or sweet potatoes instead of opting for white rice and regular potatoes is also recommended as a more nutritional choice.

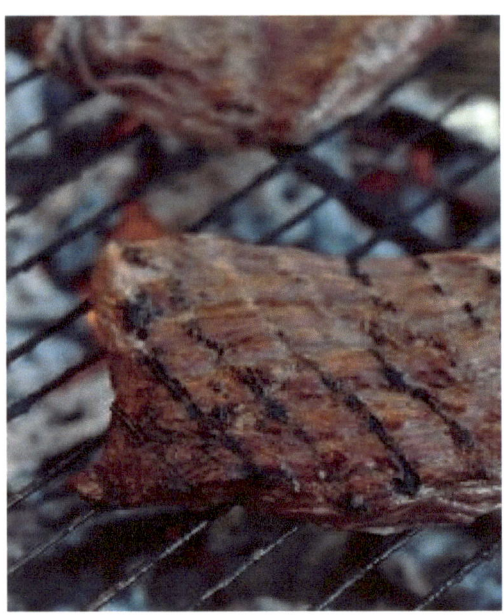

Chapter 3:

Start With What You Eat

Synopsis

When a person is first diagnosed with the medical condition called diabetes, it may seem really like the end of the world as they know it, but this is not necessarily so.

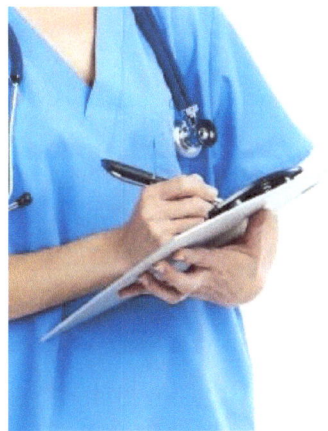

Your Diet

With some careful life changing adjustments which is mainly focused on the diet and a suitable exercise program, the diabetic can lead a healthy and wholesome life.

As with all other conditions be it medical or otherwise keeping a healthy diet plan and a good and suitable exercise regiment will usually bring forth the desired effects of a healthy body and mind. However for the diabetic there maybe some further concessions that needs to be made.

Diabetics are usually advised not to consume any while foods and to watch their intake of carbs carefully and on a regular basis. However the practice of eating apples has been found to help reduce the body's need for insulin as apples contain pectin which helps the body to detoxify.

Another fruit that is often recommended as suitable for diabetics is the pomegranate. The sugar content in the fruit does not in any way effect the blood sugar in a diabetic patient and it also decreases the risk of atherosclerosis.

As for spices, it has been noted that cinnamon and garlic are very good for diabetic patients to include in their daily diet plan. The cinnamon contains MHCP which gives fat cells new life and also helps these cells to respond better to insulin while getting rid of the glucose in the blood. The garlic contributes to keeping diabetes under control by regulating and controlling the blood sugar levels when necessary.

Oatmeal is another good item to include in the dietary plan of a diabetic patient. Considered a good crab the fiber makeup of this item allows good digestion and keeps the blood sugar levels stable.

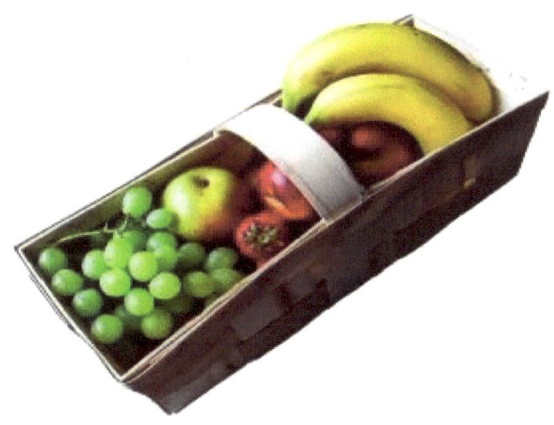

Chapter 4:

Nutrition That Cuts Out The Sugar

Synopsis

Cutting out sugar altogether may be a rather drastic measure, but if there is a diabetic medical condition than this is certainly not an option but it is a necessity. However all is not lost as there are ways to cut out the sugar content of a food item without making the said item tasteless or boring.

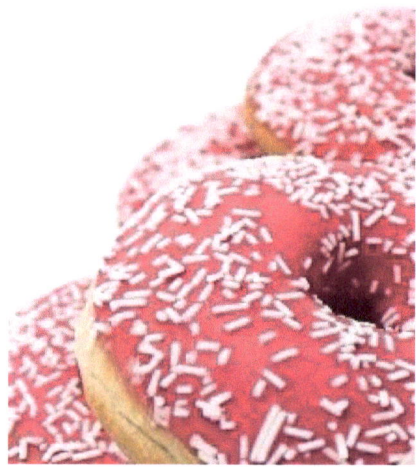

Cutting The Sugar

For breakfast choices such as cereal opting to add cinnamon, dried berries, apricots or any other dried fruits will help to bring about a natural sweetened flavor that would be better for the blood sugar levels of a diabetic patient. Another trick that can be used when trying to decrease or eliminate the use of sugar, is using a raspberry or strawberry homemade sauce on waffles and pancakes instead of sweetened syrup or a dusting of sugar.

Whenever possible substitute sugar for fruit purees as these contain natural sugar and is also a better alternative for a diabetic patient. This is especially useful when there are recipes that call for the adding of one or more cups of sugar as their measurements for ingredients.

When it comes to preparing vegetable dishes combining some sweeter vegetables with other strong flavored one will help to give off a hint of sweetness which is not only pleasant but also help to enhance the overall taste of the dish.

These may include a combination of carrots with ginger, mashed sweet potatoes with cinnamon, spinach with nutmeg and any other combination that the individual may find interesting and pleasing.

When it comes to purchasing pre prepared food items sourcing for the ones with accurate labeling will allow the diabetic patient to make informed decisions and purchase products that don't have high sugar content or at the very least have artificial sweeteners. It is possible to eventually cut out sugar altogether if some effort is made to do so gradually and not all at once.

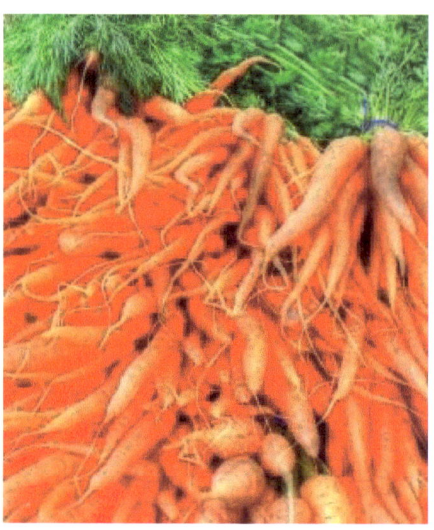

Chapter 5:

Dining Out For Diabetics

Synopsis

Besides the daily doses of insulin and a good exercise regiment, all food intake needs to be carefully monitored for a diabetic patient. All these efforts are to help control the blood glucose levels, thus the need to be extra careful.

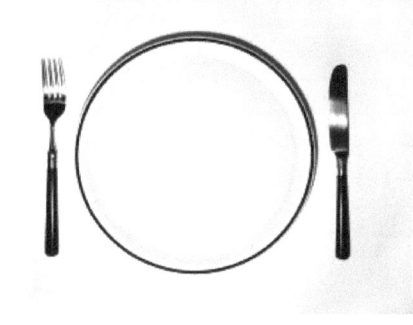

Dining Out

Eating out is no exception to these rules and it can be done in an enjoyable manner with a little bit of effort and care on the part of the diabetic patient.

There are many restaurants today that offer healthy food choices for the more discerning customers. These customers may include those who want to keep their cholesterol levels under control; some may be watching their calorie intakes while others may be interested in simply eating healthy to stay healthy.

It is easy to find restaurants that provide for all the healthy needs of a wide range of customers. Finding salads, fish, vegetables, baked or broiled goods and whole grain bread on a menu is not uncommon as most people today often opt for these choices. There are also establishments that design their menus to clearly show the calorie and fat content on their menus.

There are also restaurants that offer foods lower in cholesterol, fat and sodium and while being higher in fiber. Reduced calorie salad dressings, low fat or fat free milk and salt substitutes are also popularly offered at many restaurants today. Some restaurants will also give the customers several alternative preparation styles which may include the healthier broiled style instead of fried, skinless chicken and lean cuts of meat as opposed to the unhealthier versions which are so popularly enjoyed by the masses.

Another attractive feature is that most of these restaurants do no charge anything extra for such slight changes in the menu contents or preparations and in fact go out of their way to accommodate customers who are health conscious.

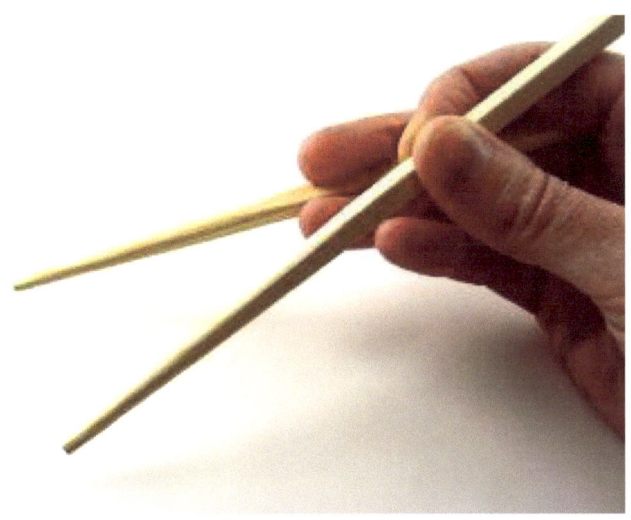

Chapter 6:

Natural Remedy To Control Sugar Levels

Synopsis

This is a disease that develops due to the problem with the hormone insulin produced by the pancreas. When this process is disrupted due to abnormalities there is insufficient control of the glucose in the blood and how much is absorbed into the cells. However there are some medical and home remedies that can be explored to control this negativity within the body.

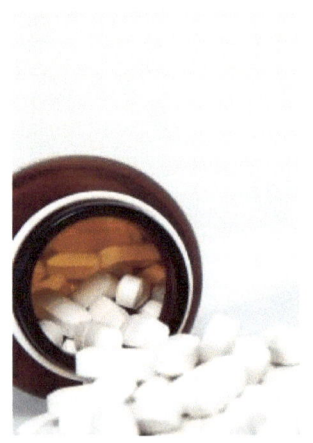

Natural Sugar Control

The following are some recommendations of home remedies that should be explored in the quest to limit the problems diabetics face:

Taking Alpha lipoid acid helps to control the sugar level in the blood and it is considered one of the elite, multipurpose antioxidants.

Taking 400mcg a day of chromium picolinate assists insulin in helping to keep the sugar levels in the body low. The chromium picolinate keeps the blood sugar level through proper insulin usage.

Taking garlic is also another very effective way of helping the circulation and regulars the sugar level. These come in convenient capsules to ensure easier consumption.

500mg of L-glutamine and taurine a day will help to reduce the sugar cravings and help to release the insulin more effectively. This is especially useful for those who have serious trouble controlling their sweet tooth tendencies.

Huckleberry has been known to promote the production of insulin in the body when taken according to prescribed amounts. The natural remedy is also quite pleasant to consume.

A concoction of tea and kidney beans, white beans, navy beans, lima beans and northern beans does help to remove the toxin from the pancreas.

There are several other natural remedies that are used to control the blood sugar levels in diabetics, however anyone of these should be taken with either medical approval or at the very least with some expert advice and in depth knowledge of the disease.

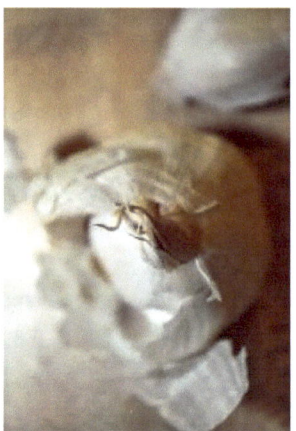

Chapter 7:

Root Vegetables And Fruits For Diabetics

Synopsis

Due to the various health problems that can occur in the body of a diabetic patient, there is a need to be rather careful with the diet plan adopted on a daily basis.

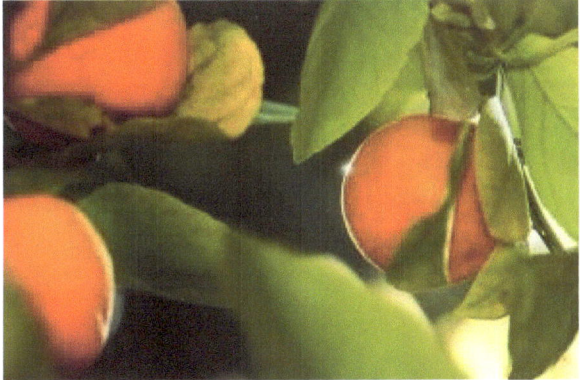

Fruits And Veggies

Any food intake needs to be done with some level of discernment to ensure its suitability for the diabetic patient. All diabetic need to ensure they adhere to a very balanced diet which is rich with vitamins and minerals, and the proteins in foods, carbs and fats also should be of an acceptable level.

Root vegetables and fruits have been accepted as a great source of vitamins and minerals as well as fiber which is instrumental in decreasing the chances of heart attack and stroke occurring possibilities. These root vegetables and fruits usually help to offset any side effects the disturbed blood sugar level causes. These side effects are likely to cause heart attacks and blindness if not controlled effectively by the regulating ingredients of vitamins and minerals derived from the root vegetable and fruits.

However it should be noted that consuming the root vegetables and fruits as a combination with other food items that are deemed suitable for a diabetic's consumption, is definitely better that consuming them as standalone items in the form of snacks. This is because when these are consumed along with other foods the chemical reactions will allow all the vitamins and the minerals to be better absorbed in the body system thereby ensuring controlled blood sugar levels. However when consumed as standalone items in the form of snacks the blood sugar levels are like to be high as the absorption levels become distorted and less that optimum. Therefore an important point to always consider is to ensure whatever food consumed should be done in a combination that allows the absorption levels to be suitable for the diabetic system to accept.

Wrapping Up

It is a fact that diabetics will face challenges and obstacles in their life due to their disease. With proper care for yourself your life could be much better though. Eating correctly and sticking to certain diets will surely have you feeling great.

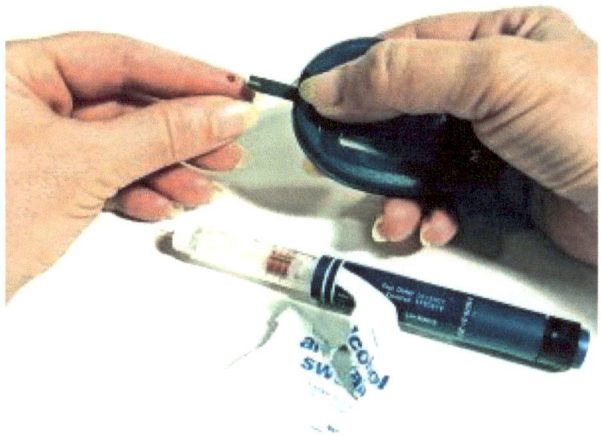